Chapter 1: Introduction to Acetylcholine

Overview of Acetylcholine (ACh) and Its Significance in the Body

Acetylcholine (ACh) is one of the most critical neurotransmitters in the human body, playing a pivotal role in various physiological processes. As the first neurotransmitter identified, ACh has garnered significant attention from researchers and healthcare professionals alike. This organic compound, classified as an ester of acetic acid and choline, is synthesized in nerve terminals and released into the synaptic cleft to facilitate communication between neurons and between neurons and muscles.

The significance of acetylcholine extends beyond mere neurotransmission. It is involved in a multitude of functions, including but not limited to muscle contraction, modulation of heart rate, regulation of sleep-wake cycles, and enhancement of cognitive functions such as memory and learning. Understanding ACh's diverse roles provides insight into its impact on both physical health and mental well-being.

Moreover, ACh serves as a critical mediator in the autonomic nervous system, influencing both the sympathetic and parasympathetic branches. Its ability to promote parasympathetic responses, such as lowering heart rate and stimulating digestion, underscores its importance in maintaining homeostasis within the body.

Historical Context and Discovery of Acetylcholine

The discovery of acetylcholine dates back to the late 19th century, when scientists began exploring the biochemical mechanisms underlying nerve impulses. In 1921, the German physiologist Otto Loewi made a groundbreaking contribution to neuroscience by demonstrating that nerve signals could be transmitted through chemical means. His famous experiment involved stimulating the vagus nerve of a frog's heart, which subsequently slowed the heart rate. When he collected the fluid from this heart and applied it to a second heart, it also slowed, confirming the presence of a chemical messenger.

Loewi identified this substance as acetylcholine, marking a significant milestone in the understanding of neurotransmission. For this discovery, he was awarded the Nobel Prize in Physiology or Medicine in 1936, along with his colleague Sir Henry Dale, who contributed to the study of ACh and its physiological effects.

Since its discovery, research into acetylcholine has expanded, revealing its integral role in both the central nervous system (CNS) and peripheral nervous system (PNS). The ongoing study of ACh has provided valuable insights into various neurological disorders, including Alzheimer's disease, myasthenia gravis, and Parkinson's disease, where disturbances in ACh production and function can lead to significant health challenges.

As we delve deeper into the complex world of acetylcholine, it becomes increasingly clear that mastering its production and availability is essential for enhancing health and well-being. This book aims to unravel the intricacies of ACh, exploring its synthesis, receptor interactions, and the factors that influence its availability in the body. By understanding acetylcholine more comprehensively, we can unlock its potential for improving cognitive function, physical performance, and overall quality of life.

Conclusion of Chapter 1

In summary, acetylcholine is a vital neurotransmitter with a rich history and extensive significance in the human body. The groundbreaking discoveries of early researchers laid the foundation for our current understanding of ACh's role in health and disease. As we proceed to the next chapters, we will explore the multifaceted functions of acetylcholine, its synthesis pathways, and the myriad factors that affect its production and availability, paving the way for effective strategies to enhance this crucial neurotransmitter's presence in our lives.

Chapter 2: The Role of Acetylcholine in the Nervous System

Understanding Neurotransmission and Synaptic Function

Acetylcholine (ACh) is a crucial neurotransmitter that facilitates communication within the nervous system. Neurotransmission, the process by which neurons send messages to each other, occurs at synapses—specialized junctions where neuronal signals are transmitted. When an electrical impulse, or action potential, reaches the end of a neuron (the presynaptic terminal), it triggers the release of ACh into the synaptic cleft.

Once in the cleft, ACh binds to specific receptors on the postsynaptic neuron, leading to a cascade of physiological responses. This binding opens ion channels, resulting in depolarization of the postsynaptic membrane and the initiation of a new action potential, thus continuing the transmission of the signal. This process highlights the importance of ACh in maintaining communication between neurons, ultimately influencing various bodily functions such as muscle movement, heart rate, and cognitive processes.

The efficiency and precision of neurotransmission depend on several factors, including the synthesis and release of ACh, receptor availability, and the termination of the signal. Acetylcholinesterase, an enzyme located in the synaptic cleft, breaks down ACh into acetate and choline, terminating its action and ensuring that signals are not inappropriately prolonged. This intricate balance of synthesis, release, receptor activation, and degradation is essential for the proper functioning of the nervous system.

The Role of Acetylcholine in the Central and Peripheral Nervous Systems

In the central nervous system (CNS), acetylcholine is instrumental in modulating various cognitive functions, including attention, learning, and memory. Cholinergic neurons, which produce ACh, are primarily located in regions such as the basal forebrain and brainstem. From these areas, they project to key regions involved in cognition, including the hippocampus and cortex. Research indicates that ACh plays a vital role in enhancing synaptic plasticity—the ability of synapses to strengthen or weaken over time, which is crucial for learning and memory formation.

Dysregulation of acetylcholine in the CNS is associated with several neurological disorders. For instance, Alzheimer's disease is characterized by a significant loss of cholinergic neurons, leading to cognitive decline and memory impairment. Thus, understanding and enhancing ACh signaling in the CNS is a focal point of therapeutic strategies aimed at improving cognitive function in neurodegenerative diseases.

In the peripheral nervous system (PNS), acetylcholine is essential for neuromuscular transmission. When a motor neuron is activated, ACh is released at the neuromuscular junction, where it binds to nicotinic receptors on the muscle fibers. This binding causes muscle contraction, allowing for voluntary movements. The role of ACh in muscle function highlights its significance in physical performance and motor control.

Additionally, ACh is a key player in the autonomic nervous system, which regulates involuntary bodily functions. In the parasympathetic branch, ACh promotes "rest and digest" responses, such as slowing the heart rate and stimulating digestive processes. Conversely, in the sympathetic branch, while ACh has a less direct role, it is involved in the modulation of responses to stress and emergency situations.

Conclusion of Chapter 2

In conclusion, acetylcholine is a fundamental neurotransmitter that plays critical roles in both the central and peripheral nervous systems. Its involvement in neurotransmission and synaptic function is vital for effective communication between neurons, influencing cognitive function and muscle activity. Understanding the multifaceted roles of ACh not only sheds light on the complexities of the nervous system but also underscores the importance of maintaining optimal ACh levels for overall health. As we advance through this book, we will explore the synthesis of acetylcholine, factors affecting its production, and strategies for enhancing its availability, ultimately aiming to master this crucial neurotransmitter for improved well-being and performance.

Chapter 3: Acetylcholine Synthesis
Biochemical Pathways of Acetylcholine Synthesis

The synthesis of acetylcholine (ACh) is a finely tuned biochemical process that occurs primarily in cholinergic neurons. This process begins with the uptake of choline, a key precursor derived from dietary sources and the breakdown of phospholipids in the cell membrane. Choline is transported into the neuron via a high-affinity choline transporter (CHT), where it enters the cytoplasm.

Once inside the neuron, choline undergoes a two-step enzymatic reaction to form ACh. The first step involves the enzyme choline acetyltransferase (ChAT), which catalyzes the transfer of an acetyl group from acetyl-CoA to choline, producing acetylcholine and coenzyme A (CoA) as a byproduct. This reaction is critical because it links the metabolic pathway of energy production (via acetyl-CoA, derived from carbohydrates, fats, and proteins) to the neurotransmitter synthesis.

The newly synthesized ACh is then stored in synaptic vesicles within the presynaptic terminal, ready to be released into the synaptic cleft when an action potential arrives. This storage is essential for efficient neurotransmission, as it allows for rapid release of ACh in response to neuronal signaling.

Key Enzymes Involved: Choline Acetyltransferase and Acetylcholinesterase

Choline Acetyltransferase (ChAT)

Choline acetyltransferase is the key enzyme responsible for the synthesis of acetylcholine. It is primarily found in cholinergic neurons and is vital for the production of ACh. The activity of ChAT can be influenced by various factors, including the availability of choline and acetyl-CoA, as well as the overall metabolic state of the neuron.

Understanding ChAT's role is essential not only for grasping ACh synthesis but also for exploring potential therapeutic targets in conditions associated with cholinergic dysfunction. For example, in neurodegenerative diseases such as Alzheimer's, where cholinergic neuron loss occurs, increasing ChAT activity may help enhance ACh levels and improve cognitive function.

Acetylcholinesterase (AChE)

Once ACh is released into the synaptic cleft and has performed its function of neurotransmission, it must be rapidly degraded to prevent excessive stimulation of the postsynaptic receptor. This degradation is carried out by acetylcholinesterase, an enzyme that hydrolyzes ACh into choline and acetate. This process is crucial for terminating the signal and ensuring that the synapse can be reset for subsequent neurotransmission.

AChE plays a significant role in regulating the duration and intensity of ACh signaling. Inhibition of AChE, through pharmacological agents known as acetylcholinesterase inhibitors, can prolong the action of ACh at the synapse. This mechanism is leveraged in the treatment of conditions such as Alzheimer's disease and myasthenia gravis, where enhanced cholinergic transmission is beneficial.

The balance between the synthesis of ACh by ChAT and its breakdown by AChE is fundamental to maintaining optimal neurotransmission. Disruptions in this balance can lead to various neurological and psychiatric disorders, highlighting the importance of understanding these enzymes and their regulation.

Conclusion of Chapter 3

In summary, the synthesis of acetylcholine is a complex biochemical process involving the uptake of choline and its conversion into ACh through the action of choline acetyltransferase. The subsequent release and degradation of ACh by acetylcholinesterase ensure that neurotransmission is finely regulated. Understanding these pathways and the key enzymes involved not only provides insight into the fundamental workings of the nervous system but also opens avenues for therapeutic interventions aimed at enhancing cholinergic function. In the following chapters, we will explore the various factors that influence ACh production, including nutritional aspects and genetic determinants, paving the way for strategies to optimize acetylcholine levels for better health and cognitive function.

Chapter 4: Factors Affecting Acetylcholine Production

Nutritional Influences: Choline Sources and Metabolism

Choline is an essential nutrient that serves as a precursor for the synthesis of acetylcholine (ACh), making its availability a crucial factor in ACh production. The body cannot produce sufficient choline on its own; therefore, dietary intake plays a vital role in maintaining adequate levels of this neurotransmitter. Choline is found in various food sources, primarily those high in phospholipids, such as egg yolks, liver, fish, poultry, dairy products, and certain nuts and seeds.

The bioavailability of choline from these food sources can vary. For instance, choline from eggs is highly bioavailable, meaning it is easily absorbed and utilized by the body. Conversely, choline from plant sources, such as soybeans and broccoli, is less efficiently absorbed. Furthermore, the form of choline consumed—whether as free choline, phosphatidylcholine, or sphingomyelin—can influence its metabolism and utilization for ACh synthesis.

The metabolism of choline in the body is also significant. Once ingested, choline undergoes several metabolic processes. In the liver, it can be converted to phosphatidylcholine, a major component of cell membranes, or it can be transported to the brain where it is used for ACh synthesis. Factors such as gut microbiota composition and overall metabolic health can impact how effectively choline is processed and utilized, emphasizing the importance of a balanced diet rich in essential nutrients.

In addition to choline, other nutrients play supporting roles in ACh synthesis. B vitamins, particularly B6, B12, and folate, are important co-factors in the metabolic pathways that convert choline into ACh. Deficiencies in these vitamins can lead to impaired ACh synthesis and subsequent neurological effects.

Impact of Genetics on ACh Synthesis

Genetic factors also significantly influence acetylcholine production and availability. Variations in genes associated with the enzymes involved in ACh synthesis and degradation can affect individual capacity to produce and regulate this neurotransmitter. For instance, polymorphisms in the gene encoding for choline acetyltransferase (ChAT) may lead to variations in the efficiency of ACh synthesis, potentially impacting cognitive function and muscle control.

Research has shown that certain genetic predispositions can influence choline metabolism. Individuals with specific genetic variations may have different needs for dietary choline or may metabolize choline at different rates. Understanding these genetic factors is critical for developing personalized dietary recommendations that support optimal ACh production.

Moreover, the interaction between genetics and environment can further complicate ACh synthesis. For example, a person with a genetic predisposition for reduced ACh synthesis may experience exacerbated effects if their diet is also low in choline. This interplay underscores the importance of considering both genetic background and lifestyle factors when evaluating ACh availability.

Conclusion of Chapter 4

In summary, both nutritional influences and genetic factors play crucial roles in acetylcholine production and availability. A well-rounded diet rich in choline and supportive nutrients is essential for maintaining optimal ACh levels, while genetic variations can impact individual responses to dietary intake and the efficiency of neurotransmitter synthesis. Understanding these factors provides a foundation for developing strategies to enhance acetylcholine availability, which is vital for cognitive function, muscle control, and overall health. As we move forward in this book, we will explore the various receptors for acetylcholine and their mechanisms of action, further elucidating the intricate balance required for effective neurotransmission.

Chapter 5: Acetylcholine Receptors

Types of Acetylcholine Receptors: Nicotinic and Muscarinic

Acetylcholine exerts its effects on target cells through two main types of receptors: nicotinic receptors and muscarinic receptors. Each receptor type plays a distinct role in mediating the physiological effects of ACh across various tissues and systems.

Nicotinic Receptors

Nicotinic acetylcholine receptors (nAChRs) are ionotropic receptors, meaning they form ion channels that open in response to acetylcholine binding. These receptors are primarily found at the neuromuscular junction in skeletal muscle, as well as in the central and peripheral nervous systems.

When ACh binds to nAChRs, it causes a conformational change in the receptor that opens the ion channel, allowing the influx of sodium ions (Na+) and, in some cases, calcium ions (Ca2+) into the cell. This influx depolarizes the cell membrane, leading to excitatory responses such as muscle contraction or neuronal firing.

Nicotinic receptors are characterized by their rapid response and short duration of action, making them essential for immediate physiological responses. For example, in skeletal muscle, the activation of nAChRs leads to muscle contraction, while in the autonomic ganglia, they facilitate synaptic transmission between pre- and post-ganglionic neurons.

Muscarinic Receptors

Muscarinic acetylcholine receptors (mAChRs), on the other hand, are G protein-coupled receptors (GPCRs) that mediate slower, longer-lasting responses. They are widely distributed throughout the central nervous system and in various peripheral tissues, including the heart, smooth muscle, and glands.

When ACh binds to mAChRs, it activates intracellular G proteins that can either stimulate or inhibit various signaling pathways depending on the specific receptor subtype involved (M1, M2, M3, M4, and M5). For example:

- **M1 receptors** are primarily found in the CNS and are involved in cognitive processes and memory.
- **M2 receptors** are located in the heart, where their activation leads to decreased heart rate and reduced contractility.
- **M3 receptors** are found in smooth muscle and glands, promoting contraction in smooth muscle and secretion in exocrine glands.

The versatility of muscarinic receptors allows ACh to influence a wide array of physiological functions, from modulating heart rate to regulating glandular secretion.

Mechanisms of Receptor Activation and Signal Transduction

The activation of both nicotinic and muscarinic receptors by acetylcholine initiates complex signaling cascades that lead to various cellular responses. Understanding these mechanisms is crucial for mastering acetylcholine's role in health and disease.

Nicotinic Receptor Activation

The mechanism of nicotinic receptor activation is relatively straightforward. Upon binding of ACh, the receptor undergoes a conformational change, opening the ion channel and allowing ions to flow into the cell. This rapid influx of sodium ions causes depolarization, leading to an action potential in neurons or muscle contraction in muscle fibers.

In addition to the direct effects on ion flow, nicotinic receptors can also engage in more complex signaling pathways. For instance, the influx of calcium ions through nAChRs can activate intracellular signaling cascades that lead to changes in gene expression and cellular function, contributing to neuroplasticity and muscle adaptation.

Muscarinic Receptor Signal Transduction

The activation of muscarinic receptors involves more intricate signaling mechanisms. When ACh binds to an mAChR, the associated G protein is activated, leading to the dissociation of its subunits. The activated G protein can then influence various effector proteins, including enzymes and ion channels.

For example, the activation of M2 receptors in the heart inhibits adenylate cyclase, reducing the production of cyclic AMP (cAMP) and leading to decreased heart rate. Conversely, the activation of M3 receptors stimulates phospholipase C, which increases inositol triphosphate (IP3) and diacylglycerol (DAG) levels, leading to increased intracellular calcium and muscle contraction.

These diverse signaling pathways enable ACh to regulate a wide range of physiological processes, emphasizing the importance of receptor type and context in mediating ACh's effects.

Conclusion of Chapter 5

In conclusion, acetylcholine receptors—both nicotinic and muscarinic—play critical roles in the function of the nervous system and beyond. Understanding the distinct characteristics of these receptors, their activation mechanisms, and the resulting signal transduction pathways is essential for mastering the complexities of acetylcholine's effects on the body. As we proceed to the next chapters, we will explore the relationship between acetylcholine and cognitive function, muscle activity, and other critical aspects of health, further illuminating the multifaceted role of this vital neurotransmitter.

Chapter 6: Acetylcholine and Cognitive Function
The Relationship Between Acetylcholine and Memory

Acetylcholine (ACh) plays a pivotal role in cognitive functions, particularly memory formation and retrieval. Research has established a strong link between cholinergic signaling and various types of memory, including working memory, spatial memory, and long-term memory. The brain regions most associated with ACh's role in cognition include the hippocampus, cortex, and basal forebrain, where cholinergic neurons are densely located.

The hippocampus, known for its critical involvement in learning and memory processes, is particularly sensitive to changes in ACh levels. Increased ACh availability has been shown to enhance synaptic plasticity, a fundamental mechanism underlying learning and memory. In experimental studies, the infusion of ACh into the hippocampus has been found to improve performance on memory tasks, suggesting that adequate levels of this neurotransmitter are necessary for optimal cognitive function.

Conversely, deficits in ACh signaling are closely associated with memory impairments. Conditions such as Alzheimer's disease, characterized by significant loss of cholinergic neurons, lead to pronounced memory deficits and cognitive decline. This relationship emphasizes the importance of maintaining healthy ACh levels for preserving cognitive functions throughout life.

ACh's Role in Learning and Neuroplasticity

Beyond its role in memory, acetylcholine is also crucial for learning processes and neuroplasticity—the brain's ability to reorganize and adapt itself in response to new information or experiences. ACh facilitates the modulation of synaptic strength, enabling the formation of new neural connections that underpin learning.

Cholinergic activity is particularly important during the initial stages of learning when new information is being encoded. The presence of ACh enhances the plasticity of synapses, making them more responsive to incoming signals. This effect is mediated through ACh's interaction with both nicotinic and muscarinic receptors, which can influence various intracellular signaling pathways.

In addition to promoting synaptic plasticity, ACh is involved in the consolidation of memories. During sleep, particularly during rapid eye movement (REM) sleep, ACh levels fluctuate, suggesting its role in memory consolidation and the integration of new experiences. The intricate interplay between ACh and sleep underscores the importance of a well-regulated cholinergic system for optimal cognitive health.

Research has also indicated that physical exercise can enhance ACh signaling and promote neuroplasticity. Aerobic activity has been shown to increase the expression of choline acetyltransferase, the enzyme responsible for synthesizing ACh, thereby boosting ACh levels in the brain. This connection highlights the potential of lifestyle interventions to positively influence cognitive function through modulation of acetylcholine production.

Implications for Cognitive Health and Disorders

Understanding the relationship between acetylcholine and cognitive function has significant implications for the prevention and treatment of cognitive disorders. Strategies aimed at enhancing ACh availability could offer therapeutic benefits for individuals at risk of or already experiencing cognitive decline.

For example, pharmacological interventions, such as acetylcholinesterase inhibitors, are already used in the management of Alzheimer's disease to increase the levels of ACh in the brain. Additionally, lifestyle factors such as diet, exercise, and cognitive training programs that enhance ACh production and signaling may serve as preventative measures against cognitive decline.

Moreover, ongoing research into the mechanisms by which ACh influences cognitive processes may yield novel therapeutic targets for improving cognitive function in aging populations and individuals with neurodegenerative diseases.

Conclusion of Chapter 6

In summary, acetylcholine is integral to cognitive function, influencing memory, learning, and neuroplasticity. The interplay between ACh levels and cognitive processes underscores the importance of maintaining healthy cholinergic signaling for optimal brain health. As we continue through this book, we will explore the role of acetylcholine in muscle function, further illustrating the wide-ranging effects of this vital neurotransmitter on both mental and physical performance.

Chapter 7: Acetylcholine in Muscle Function

ACh's Role in Neuromuscular Junctions

Acetylcholine (ACh) is crucial for the proper functioning of the neuromuscular junction (NMJ), the synapse between a motor neuron and a muscle fiber. This specialized connection is essential for initiating muscle contraction, enabling voluntary movements and supporting various physiological functions, from walking to breathing.

When a motor neuron is activated, an action potential travels down the axon and reaches the presynaptic terminal at the NMJ. This electrical signal triggers the influx of calcium ions (Ca^{2+}) into the neuron, promoting the release of ACh from synaptic vesicles into the synaptic cleft. ACh then diffuses across the cleft and binds to nicotinic acetylcholine receptors (nAChRs) located on the muscle fiber's postsynaptic membrane.

The binding of ACh to these receptors opens ion channels, allowing sodium ions (Na^+) to flow into the muscle cell, leading to depolarization of the membrane. If the depolarization reaches a threshold, it generates an action potential in the muscle fiber, which ultimately triggers the release of calcium from the sarcoplasmic reticulum. This calcium release initiates the sliding filament mechanism of muscle contraction, allowing the muscle to shorten and generate force.

Implications for Muscle Contraction and Motor Control

The precise regulation of ACh at the NMJ is critical for effective muscle contraction and motor control. A deficiency in ACh production or receptor sensitivity can lead to various neuromuscular disorders, characterized by muscle weakness and fatigue. Conditions such as myasthenia gravis involve the production of antibodies that block or destroy nAChRs, impairing ACh binding and resulting in compromised muscle function.

Conversely, excessive ACh activity can lead to muscle spasms and cramps. This balance is vital for maintaining normal muscle tone and coordination during movement. The body relies on a feedback mechanism that involves the modulation of ACh release, receptor sensitivity, and the action of acetylcholinesterase (AChE) to break down excess ACh in the synaptic cleft.

The role of ACh extends beyond the NMJ to influence various aspects of muscle physiology, including endurance and recovery. Studies have shown that cholinergic signaling can impact muscle metabolism, promoting adaptations in muscle fibers that enhance their performance during physical activity. Adequate ACh levels are necessary for optimizing muscle function, particularly in high-demand situations like exercise.

The Interplay Between ACh and Other Factors in Muscle Function

Several factors influence the availability and effectiveness of ACh at the NMJ, including nutritional status, exercise, and overall health. Nutrients like choline, as discussed in earlier chapters, are vital for ACh synthesis, while factors such as hydration, electrolyte balance, and overall energy availability can impact neuromuscular function.

Physical activity also plays a significant role in modulating ACh levels. Regular exercise has been shown to enhance ACh synthesis and release, contributing to improved muscle performance and coordination. Additionally, resistance training can promote adaptations in the NMJ, increasing the efficiency of ACh signaling and muscle contraction.

Stress and fatigue can negatively impact ACh function and receptor sensitivity, leading to diminished muscle performance. Implementing stress management strategies and ensuring adequate rest and recovery can help maintain healthy ACh levels and optimal muscle function.

Conclusion of Chapter 7

In summary, acetylcholine is essential for muscle function, particularly at the neuromuscular junction, where it facilitates the transmission of signals from motor neurons to muscle fibers. Understanding the role of ACh in muscle contraction and motor control highlights its importance not only for voluntary movements but also for overall physical performance and health.

As we progress in this book, we will examine how aging affects acetylcholine levels and its implications for muscle function and cognitive health, further emphasizing the interconnectedness of ACh's role across various bodily systems.

Chapter 8: The Impact of Age on Acetylcholine Levels
Changes in ACh Production with Aging

As individuals age, there are significant changes in the production and availability of acetylcholine (ACh) that can affect cognitive and physical health. Research has consistently shown that cholinergic neurons, which are responsible for the synthesis and release of ACh, decline in number and function with age. This decline leads to reduced ACh production, impacting various physiological processes, particularly in the central nervous system.

The basal forebrain, a key area rich in cholinergic neurons, is particularly affected by aging. Studies indicate that the loss of these neurons correlates with declines in cognitive function, including memory, attention, and executive functions. This decline is thought to be related to the neurotransmitter's crucial role in learning and memory processes, as highlighted in previous chapters.

Furthermore, age-related changes in ACh metabolism and receptor sensitivity can exacerbate the effects of reduced ACh production. The efficiency of nicotinic and muscarinic receptors may decline, leading to impaired synaptic transmission and reduced neural plasticity. This situation can create a feedback loop where decreased receptor function leads to further reductions in ACh signaling.

Neurodegenerative Diseases Related to ACh Deficiency

The decline in ACh production and function with aging is particularly concerning given its association with neurodegenerative diseases, most notably Alzheimer's disease. Alzheimer's is characterized by the progressive degeneration of cholinergic neurons, particularly in the basal forebrain, which contributes significantly to the cognitive decline experienced by patients.

The cholinergic hypothesis of Alzheimer's disease posits that the loss of ACh-producing neurons and the resultant decrease in ACh levels are fundamental to the cognitive deficits seen in this condition. Clinical trials have demonstrated that enhancing cholinergic activity through acetylcholinesterase inhibitors can lead to modest improvements in cognitive function, underscoring the importance of ACh in maintaining cognitive health.

In addition to Alzheimer's, other neurodegenerative diseases, such as Parkinson's disease and Huntington's disease, also exhibit cholinergic dysfunction. In these conditions, the interplay between ACh and other neurotransmitters becomes disrupted, leading to a complex network of deficits that contribute to motor and cognitive impairments.

Moreover, age-related changes in ACh are not limited to neurodegenerative diseases. Conditions such as vascular dementia, where blood flow to the brain is compromised, can also affect ACh levels and function. The decline in ACh can exacerbate the symptoms of these conditions, leading to significant challenges in managing cognitive health as individuals age.

Implications for Aging and Cognitive Health

Understanding the impact of aging on ACh levels emphasizes the importance of strategies aimed at preserving cholinergic function throughout life. Lifestyle interventions, including regular physical activity, cognitive training, and a nutrient-rich diet, can potentially help mitigate the age-related decline in ACh production and function.

Engaging in activities that promote neuroplasticity—such as learning new skills, participating in social interactions, and exercising—may stimulate the cholinergic system and enhance cognitive resilience. Additionally, ensuring adequate intake of choline-rich foods, as well as other nutrients involved in ACh synthesis, can support optimal levels of this vital neurotransmitter.

Emerging research into pharmacological interventions that target ACh production and receptor sensitivity holds promise for addressing age-related cognitive decline. Such approaches may complement lifestyle strategies, providing a multifaceted approach to maintaining cognitive health as individuals age.

Conclusion of Chapter 8

In conclusion, the aging process significantly impacts acetylcholine production and availability, leading to cognitive and physical health challenges. The decline of cholinergic neurons and the resultant reduction in ACh levels are closely associated with neurodegenerative diseases, highlighting the importance of understanding and addressing these changes.

As we progress through this book, we will explore the connections between acetylcholine and mental health, examining how ACh levels influence mood and stress responses. This understanding will further illuminate the intricate role of ACh in overall health and well-being.

Chapter 9: Acetylcholine and Mental Health

The Connection Between ACh Levels and Mood Disorders

Acetylcholine (ACh) has been recognized not only for its critical roles in cognitive function and muscle control but also for its significant influence on mental health. Research suggests that ACh levels can affect mood regulation, emotional stability, and overall mental well-being. Dysregulation of cholinergic signaling has been linked to several mood disorders, including depression and anxiety, underscoring the importance of maintaining healthy ACh levels for optimal mental health.

Several studies have found that individuals with depression often exhibit reduced cholinergic activity and lower levels of ACh in certain brain regions. The cholinergic system is involved in modulating neurotransmitter release, and its dysfunction can disrupt the balance of other key neurotransmitters, such as serotonin and dopamine, which play vital roles in mood regulation. This interplay suggests that restoring ACh function could have therapeutic implications for mood disorders.

Moreover, animal studies have shown that pharmacological agents that enhance cholinergic activity can lead to antidepressant-like effects. These findings support the hypothesis that increasing ACh levels may help alleviate symptoms of depression, providing a potential avenue for novel treatment strategies.

ACh's Role in Stress Response and Anxiety

Acetylcholine also plays a crucial role in the body's stress response. During periods of stress, ACh release can influence both the autonomic nervous system and the hypothalamic-pituitary-adrenal (HPA) axis, which regulates the body's reaction to stress. The cholinergic system helps to modulate the balance between the sympathetic and parasympathetic nervous systems, impacting how individuals respond to stressors.

In particular, the activation of muscarinic receptors in the brain has been shown to influence anxiety levels. Increased ACh activity can promote calmness and relaxation by facilitating parasympathetic responses, while decreased ACh availability may exacerbate feelings of anxiety. Research indicates that enhancing cholinergic function can have anxiolytic effects, making it a potential target for anxiety treatment.

Additionally, the connection between ACh and cognitive function is particularly relevant in the context of anxiety disorders. Individuals experiencing anxiety often report difficulties with concentration, memory, and decision-making, which can be attributed to dysregulated cholinergic signaling. Therefore, strategies that enhance ACh production and receptor sensitivity may improve both cognitive function and anxiety symptoms.

Implications for Mental Health Treatment

Understanding the relationship between acetylcholine and mental health opens the door for developing targeted therapeutic approaches. Enhancing cholinergic signaling through lifestyle interventions, dietary modifications, and pharmacological treatments could provide a multifaceted strategy for improving mental health.

1. **Dietary Strategies**: Incorporating choline-rich foods into the diet, such as eggs, meat, fish, and nuts, can support ACh synthesis. Omega-3 fatty acids, found in fatty fish and flaxseeds, may also play a role in promoting cholinergic function.
2. **Physical Activity**: Regular exercise has been shown to enhance ACh levels and improve mood. Engaging in aerobic activities can stimulate the release of growth factors that promote neurogenesis and cholinergic signaling.
3. **Mindfulness and Stress Reduction**: Practices such as meditation, yoga, and mindfulness-based stress reduction can help modulate the body's stress response and improve cholinergic function, potentially reducing symptoms of anxiety and depression.
4. **Pharmacological Approaches**: As discussed in previous chapters, acetylcholinesterase inhibitors are currently used in treating Alzheimer's disease and have shown potential benefits in managing mood disorders. Continued research into cholinergic agents may yield new treatment options for anxiety and depression.

Conclusion of Chapter 9

In conclusion, acetylcholine plays a vital role in mental health, influencing mood, stress response, and cognitive function. Understanding the connection between ACh levels and mood disorders highlights the importance of maintaining healthy cholinergic signaling for overall well-being. As we advance through this book, we will explore strategies for enhancing acetylcholine production, further emphasizing its significance in promoting mental health and cognitive resilience.

Chapter 10: Enhancing Acetylcholine Production
Dietary Strategies to Boost ACh Synthesis

Acetylcholine (ACh) synthesis is critically dependent on adequate levels of choline, the primary precursor for this important neurotransmitter. Consequently, dietary strategies to increase choline intake can significantly enhance ACh production. Several foods are particularly rich in choline, including:

1. **Eggs**: One of the best sources of choline, particularly in the yolk. Eggs are also versatile and easy to incorporate into various diets.
2. **Meat and Poultry**: Beef, chicken, and turkey are excellent sources of choline, providing substantial amounts per serving. Organ meats, such as liver, are especially rich in this nutrient.
3. **Fish**: Fatty fish like salmon and sardines not only provide choline but are also high in omega-3 fatty acids, which support brain health.
4. **Dairy Products**: Milk and yogurt are good sources of choline and can be beneficial for those who include dairy in their diets.
5. **Legumes and Nuts**: Foods like soybeans, lentils, and peanuts provide decent amounts of choline, making them suitable options for vegetarians and vegans.
6. **Cruciferous Vegetables**: Broccoli, Brussels sprouts, and cauliflower contain choline and are also high in fiber and other beneficial nutrients.

In addition to increasing choline-rich foods, it is essential to ensure a well-balanced diet that supports overall metabolic health. Nutrients such as B vitamins (particularly B6, B12, and folate) are also important for ACh synthesis and metabolism. A deficiency in these vitamins can impair the body's ability to produce and utilize ACh effectively.

Supplements and Their Effects on ACh Availability

While dietary intake is crucial, supplements can also play a role in enhancing ACh production and availability. Several supplements are commonly used to support cholinergic function:

1. **Choline Supplements**: Choline is available in various forms, including choline bitartrate, phosphatidylcholine, and alpha-GPC. These supplements can help increase overall choline levels in the body, thereby promoting ACh synthesis. Alpha-GPC, in particular, has been shown to effectively cross the blood-brain barrier and may enhance cognitive function.

2. **Citicoline (CDP-Choline)**: Citicoline is another supplement that can boost choline levels and has been shown to support cognitive health. It is believed to enhance the synthesis of phosphatidylcholine, a key component of cell membranes, and may also have neuroprotective effects.

3. **Acetyl-L-Carnitine**: This amino acid derivative has been associated with increased ACh levels and improved cognitive function. It may enhance mitochondrial function and support the health of cholinergic neurons.

4. **Omega-3 Fatty Acids**: While not directly related to ACh synthesis, omega-3 fatty acids have been shown to support overall brain health and may positively influence cholinergic signaling. Supplements like fish oil can help provide these essential fats.

5. **Phosphatidylserine**: This phospholipid has been linked to improved cognitive function and may help enhance ACh release at synapses. It is often used as a supplement for cognitive support.

Before beginning any supplementation regimen, it is advisable to consult with a healthcare professional, particularly for individuals with pre-existing health conditions or those taking medications.

Lifestyle Factors That Influence ACh Production

Beyond diet and supplements, various lifestyle factors can significantly impact ACh production and availability. Here are some key considerations:

1. **Exercise**: Regular physical activity has been shown to enhance ACh synthesis and release. Exercise increases blood flow to the brain and promotes neurogenesis, which can support cholinergic function. Aerobic exercise, in particular, has been associated with improvements in cognitive function and ACh signaling.
2. **Sleep**: Quality sleep is essential for overall brain health, including optimal ACh function. During sleep, particularly REM sleep, ACh levels fluctuate, influencing memory consolidation and synaptic plasticity. Establishing good sleep hygiene practices can support healthy ACh levels.
3. **Stress Management**: Chronic stress can negatively affect ACh production and receptor sensitivity. Employing stress reduction techniques such as mindfulness meditation, yoga, and deep breathing exercises can help mitigate the effects of stress and support cholinergic function.
4. **Hydration**: Adequate hydration is crucial for maintaining overall health and supporting neurotransmitter function. Dehydration can impair cognitive performance and may negatively affect ACh availability.
5. **Cognitive Engagement**: Engaging in mentally stimulating activities, such as learning new skills, playing musical instruments, or participating in social interactions, can enhance cholinergic signaling and promote neuroplasticity.

Conclusion of Chapter 10

In summary, enhancing acetylcholine production is achievable through a combination of dietary strategies, supplementation, and lifestyle modifications. By focusing on choline-rich foods, utilizing appropriate supplements, and adopting healthy lifestyle practices, individuals can optimize ACh levels and support cognitive and physical health.

As we continue through this book, we will explore pharmacological approaches to modulate acetylcholine, examining the role of cholinergic drugs and their therapeutic applications. This knowledge will further empower individuals to master acetylcholine production and availability for improved overall well-being.

Chapter 11: Pharmacological Approaches to Modulate Acetylcholine

Overview of Cholinergic Drugs and Their Uses

Pharmacological interventions targeting the cholinergic system are pivotal in managing various neurological and psychiatric disorders. Cholinergic drugs can enhance or inhibit acetylcholine (ACh) activity, depending on their mechanism of action. These drugs are classified primarily into two categories: cholinergic agonists, which mimic the effects of ACh, and cholinergic antagonists, which block the action of ACh at its receptors.

Cholinergic Agonists

Cholinergic agonists are compounds that stimulate the action of ACh at its receptors, promoting cholinergic signaling. They are used in various clinical settings, especially for conditions characterized by reduced cholinergic function. Key examples include:

1. **Pilocarpine**: A muscarinic agonist, pilocarpine is primarily used to treat glaucoma by increasing the outflow of aqueous humor, thereby reducing intraocular pressure. It is also employed in the management of dry mouth conditions (xerostomia).
2. **Bethanechol**: This drug is used to treat urinary retention by stimulating the bladder's detrusor muscle via muscarinic receptors, promoting urination.
3. **Nicotine**: A potent nicotinic agonist, nicotine is primarily known for its use in smoking cessation therapies. It acts on nicotinic receptors in the central nervous system to enhance cognitive function and reduce withdrawal symptoms.

Cholinergic Antagonists

Cholinergic antagonists, also known as anticholinergics, block the action of ACh at its receptors. They are used in various clinical scenarios, particularly where ACh's action would be detrimental. Examples include:

1. **Atropine**: Derived from the belladonna plant, atropine is used to increase heart rate in bradycardia, reduce salivation during surgery, and treat certain types of poisoning. It acts as a muscarinic antagonist, inhibiting parasympathetic effects.
2. **Scopolamine**: This anticholinergic drug is used to prevent motion sickness and nausea by blocking muscarinic receptors in the vestibular system and the vomiting center of the brain.
3. **Ipratropium**: A muscarinic antagonist used in the treatment of chronic obstructive pulmonary disease (COPD) and asthma, it helps to relax bronchial muscles and open airways.

The Role of Acetylcholinesterase Inhibitors

Acetylcholinesterase inhibitors (AChEIs) are a significant pharmacological class that increases ACh levels by preventing its breakdown in the synaptic cleft. By inhibiting the enzyme acetylcholinesterase, these drugs prolong the action of ACh at both nicotinic and muscarinic receptors. AChEIs are particularly important in the treatment of cognitive disorders and neuromuscular conditions. Key examples include:

1. **Donepezil**: Primarily used for Alzheimer's disease, donepezil enhances cholinergic neurotransmission by inhibiting acetylcholinesterase, leading to improved cognitive function and memory.
2. **Rivastigmine**: This AChEI is also indicated for Alzheimer's and Parkinson's disease dementia. It has dual inhibitory effects on both AChE and butyrylcholinesterase, further increasing ACh availability.
3. **Galantamine**: Another AChEI used to treat Alzheimer's disease, galantamine enhances cholinergic function and may also have neuroprotective properties through its action on nicotinic receptors.
4. **Pyridostigmine**: Used in the treatment of myasthenia gravis, pyridostigmine increases ACh availability at the neuromuscular junction, improving muscle strength and function.

While AChEIs can provide symptomatic relief in conditions characterized by cholinergic deficits, they are not curative. The benefits they provide can vary among individuals and may be accompanied by side effects, including gastrointestinal issues, bradycardia, and muscle cramps.

Considerations in Pharmacological Modulation of ACh

When considering pharmacological approaches to modulate ACh, it is essential to balance therapeutic benefits with potential side effects. Individual responses to cholinergic drugs can vary based on factors such as genetics, age, and overall health. Moreover, the interaction of cholinergic drugs with other medications must be carefully monitored to avoid adverse effects.

Personalized medicine approaches that consider an individual's genetic profile and lifestyle may enhance the efficacy and safety of cholinergic treatments. Research into the pharmacogenomics of cholinergic drugs may provide insights into optimizing treatment strategies for conditions linked to ACh dysregulation.

Conclusion of Chapter 11

In conclusion, pharmacological approaches to modulating acetylcholine levels play a crucial role in treating various neurological and psychiatric disorders. Cholinergic agonists and antagonists, along with acetylcholinesterase inhibitors, are integral to managing conditions associated with cholinergic dysfunction. Understanding these pharmacological options allows for targeted interventions that can enhance cognitive function, improve muscle control, and support mental health.

As we move forward in this book, we will explore the intricate relationship between acetylcholine and other neurotransmitters, emphasizing the importance of a balanced approach to neurotransmitter systems for optimal brain health and overall well-being.

Chapter 12: The Relationship Between Acetylcholine and Other Neurotransmitters

Interactions with Dopamine, Serotonin, and Norepinephrine

Acetylcholine (ACh) does not function in isolation; it is intricately connected to other neurotransmitters, particularly dopamine, serotonin, and norepinephrine. Understanding these interactions is essential for mastering the roles of ACh in both cognitive and emotional regulation, as well as its implications for various neurological and psychiatric disorders.

1. Acetylcholine and Dopamine

The relationship between ACh and dopamine is particularly notable in the context of the brain's reward system and movement control. Dopamine, produced primarily in the substantia nigra and ventral tegmental area, is critical for regulating mood, reward, and motor function.

- **Motor Control**: ACh and dopamine interact in the striatum, where they modulate the motor pathways. Dopamine facilitates motor activity, while ACh can enhance the precision of movement. In Parkinson's disease, where dopamine levels are severely depleted, the cholinergic system often becomes overactive, leading to tremors and rigidity.
- **Reward and Motivation**: The interplay between ACh and dopamine is also crucial in processes related to reward and motivation. ACh can influence dopamine release in response to rewarding stimuli, enhancing motivation and the learning associated with rewards. This interaction suggests that ACh may play a role in addiction and substance use disorders, where dopaminergic pathways are often hijacked.

2. Acetylcholine and Serotonin

Serotonin, often referred to as the "feel-good" neurotransmitter, is involved in mood regulation, sleep, and appetite control. The relationship between ACh and serotonin is complex and bidirectional.

- **Mood Regulation**: ACh has been shown to facilitate the release of serotonin in certain brain regions, thereby influencing mood and emotional responses. This interaction is significant in understanding how cholinergic dysfunction may contribute to mood disorders, such as depression and anxiety.
- **Sleep-Wake Cycle**: ACh is integral to the regulation of REM sleep, during which serotonin levels also fluctuate. The balance between these neurotransmitters is essential for maintaining healthy sleep patterns. Dysregulation in this balance may lead to sleep disorders, which often co-occur with mood disorders.

3. Acetylcholine and Norepinephrine

Norepinephrine, a neurotransmitter involved in the body's stress response, plays a significant role in attention, arousal, and the fight-or-flight response. The interaction between ACh and norepinephrine is crucial for cognitive function and alertness.

- **Attention and Focus**: ACh promotes cortical arousal and attention, while norepinephrine enhances the brain's responsiveness to stimuli. Together, they play a pivotal role in focusing attention and facilitating learning processes. This interaction is particularly important in conditions such as ADHD, where both cholinergic and noradrenergic systems may be dysfunctional.
- **Stress Response**: ACh and norepinephrine also interact in the context of stress regulation. Under stress, norepinephrine release increases, which can enhance cholinergic signaling to modulate cognitive processes. However, chronic stress may disrupt this balance, leading to impaired cognitive function and increased anxiety.

Balancing Neurotransmitter Systems for Optimal Brain Health

Understanding the interactions between ACh and other neurotransmitters emphasizes the importance of a balanced neurotransmitter system for optimal brain health. Imbalances in these systems can lead to various neurological and psychiatric conditions.

- **Holistic Approaches**: Treatment strategies aimed at restoring balance among these neurotransmitters may prove beneficial. For instance, medications that target one neurotransmitter may have secondary effects on others. Therefore, a comprehensive understanding of these interactions can guide the development of more effective treatment protocols.
- **Lifestyle Interventions**: Non-pharmacological approaches, such as diet, exercise, and stress management, can also influence the balance of neurotransmitters. Activities that promote overall brain health can help maintain optimal levels of ACh, dopamine, serotonin, and norepinephrine, supporting cognitive and emotional well-being.

Conclusion of Chapter 12

In conclusion, the intricate relationships between acetylcholine and other neurotransmitters such as dopamine, serotonin, and norepinephrine are vital for understanding the complexity of brain function and behavior. These interactions play critical roles in cognitive processes, mood regulation, and overall mental health.

As we proceed through this book, we will delve into the influence of acetylcholine on neuroplasticity, exploring its therapeutic implications for rehabilitation and recovery. This knowledge will further enhance our understanding of how to master acetylcholine production and availability for improved cognitive and emotional health.

Chapter 13: Acetylcholine and Neuroplasticity

How ACh Influences Synaptic Plasticity

Acetylcholine (ACh) plays a crucial role in synaptic plasticity, the process by which synapses strengthen or weaken over time in response to increases or decreases in their activity. This plasticity is fundamental to learning and memory, as it underlies the brain's ability to adapt and reorganize itself. ACh modulates several mechanisms involved in synaptic plasticity, including long-term potentiation (LTP) and long-term depression (LTD).

1. **Long-Term Potentiation (LTP)**: LTP is a long-lasting enhancement in synaptic strength following a high-frequency stimulation of a synapse. ACh promotes LTP in the hippocampus, a region critically involved in memory formation. When ACh binds to its receptors, it increases intracellular calcium levels, which activate signaling pathways that lead to the strengthening of synaptic connections. This process enhances the efficacy of neurotransmitter release and receptor sensitivity, facilitating improved communication between neurons.

2. **Long-Term Depression (LTD)**: In contrast, LTD is a long-lasting decrease in synaptic strength, typically occurring after low-frequency stimulation. ACh's role in LTD is less clear but is thought to involve the activation of different signaling pathways that may reduce synaptic efficacy. The balance between LTP and LTD, influenced by ACh levels, is essential for learning new information and for the removal of unnecessary synaptic connections.

Therapeutic Implications for Rehabilitation and Recovery

Understanding the role of ACh in neuroplasticity opens up exciting therapeutic avenues for rehabilitation and recovery from neurological injuries and disorders. Here are some potential implications:

1. **Cognitive Rehabilitation**: Interventions aimed at enhancing cholinergic function may improve cognitive recovery following brain injuries or strokes. By using AChE inhibitors or cholinergic agonists, it may be possible to promote neuroplasticity and enhance cognitive function in affected individuals. Cognitive training exercises, combined with pharmacological treatments, could further stimulate ACh activity and support recovery.

2. **Neurodegenerative Diseases**: In conditions like Alzheimer's disease, where cholinergic signaling is severely impaired, strategies to boost ACh availability could help mitigate cognitive decline. Research into AChE inhibitors and other cholinergic agents is ongoing, with the goal of enhancing neuroplasticity and supporting cognitive resilience in aging populations.

3. **Physical Rehabilitation**: ACh's role in synaptic plasticity also extends to motor learning and physical rehabilitation. Enhancing cholinergic signaling can improve muscle function and motor control following injury. Physical therapy programs that incorporate exercises to stimulate both muscle and cognitive function may optimize recovery outcomes.

4. **Learning and Memory Enhancement**: For individuals seeking to enhance learning and memory, interventions that promote ACh production or receptor sensitivity could provide benefits. This could involve dietary strategies, supplements, or cognitive training designed to engage and strengthen the cholinergic system.

5. **Neurofeedback and Brain Training**: Emerging technologies, such as neurofeedback and brain-computer interfaces, may harness ACh's influence on neuroplasticity to promote cognitive and motor rehabilitation. By training individuals to increase ACh activity through mental exercises, it may be possible to enhance learning outcomes and improve cognitive function.

Conclusion of Chapter 13

In conclusion, acetylcholine is a key player in the processes of synaptic plasticity, influencing both long-term potentiation and long-term depression. Understanding ACh's role in these mechanisms has significant therapeutic implications for enhancing recovery and rehabilitation in various neurological conditions.

As we continue through this book, we will explore the role of acetylcholine in sleep regulation, examining how this neurotransmitter contributes to restorative sleep and its implications for overall health and cognitive function. This knowledge will further enrich our understanding of how to master acetylcholine production and availability for optimal cognitive and physical well-being.

Chapter 14: Acetylcholine and Sleep
The Role of ACh in Sleep Regulation

Acetylcholine (ACh) plays a critical role in the regulation of sleep, particularly in the modulation of the sleep-wake cycle and the promotion of REM (rapid eye movement) sleep. ACh is one of the key neurotransmitters involved in the transition between different sleep stages and in the processes that facilitate restorative sleep.

1. **Sleep-Wake Cycle**: ACh levels fluctuate throughout the day and night, contributing to the body's circadian rhythms. During wakefulness, cholinergic activity increases, promoting alertness and cognitive function. As the body transitions into sleep, particularly REM sleep, ACh activity surges in specific brain regions, such as the pons and the basal forebrain, facilitating the onset of this critical sleep stage.

2. **REM Sleep**: REM sleep is characterized by rapid eye movements, vivid dreaming, and increased brain activity. ACh is essential for the initiation and maintenance of REM sleep, as it promotes the activity of specific brain circuits involved in this phase. The release of ACh during REM sleep has been shown to inhibit the activity of certain neurons that regulate non-REM sleep, allowing for the unique characteristics of REM to emerge.

3. **Memory Consolidation**: Sleep, particularly REM sleep, is crucial for memory consolidation—the process by which short-term memories are transformed into long-term memories. ACh's role in facilitating REM sleep suggests that it is indirectly involved in memory processing. Enhanced ACh activity during REM may contribute to the consolidation of new learning, making it a vital component of cognitive health.

Implications for Sleep Disorders and Treatment

Given ACh's integral role in sleep regulation, dysregulation of cholinergic signaling can lead to sleep disorders, such as insomnia and obstructive sleep apnea. Here are some key implications and treatment considerations:

1. **Insomnia**: Individuals with insomnia often experience disturbances in sleep architecture, including reduced REM sleep. Pharmacological approaches that enhance cholinergic activity may help improve sleep quality. Cholinergic agonists, such as certain sedatives or sleep aids, could be explored for their potential to promote REM sleep and improve overall sleep patterns.

2. **Obstructive Sleep Apnea (OSA)**: In OSA, the cessation of breathing during sleep leads to fragmented sleep and decreased REM sleep. Research into the role of ACh in airway regulation may yield insights into potential treatments. Interventions that target cholinergic signaling could improve muscle tone in the upper airway, reducing the frequency of apneic events.

3. **REM Sleep Behavior Disorder (RBD)**: In RBD, individuals act out their dreams during REM sleep due to a lack of muscle atonia, a phenomenon normally induced by cholinergic activity. Understanding the cholinergic system's involvement in REM sleep can inform treatment strategies, including the use of AChE inhibitors, which may help restore the balance of neurotransmission during sleep.

4. **Sleep Quality and Cognitive Function**: Given the strong link between sleep quality and cognitive function, interventions that enhance ACh production and signaling may indirectly support better cognitive health. Lifestyle modifications that promote good sleep hygiene, combined with dietary strategies to increase choline intake, can be beneficial for both sleep and cognitive performance.

Lifestyle Interventions to Support ACh and Sleep

In addition to pharmacological approaches, lifestyle interventions can also enhance cholinergic function and improve sleep quality. Here are some strategies to consider:

1. **Regular Sleep Schedule**: Establishing a consistent sleep routine helps regulate circadian rhythms and supports healthy ACh activity. Going to bed and waking up at the same time each day can enhance sleep quality.
2. **Physical Activity**: Regular exercise has been shown to improve sleep quality and promote healthy ACh signaling. Engaging in aerobic exercise during the day can help facilitate deeper sleep at night.
3. **Mindfulness and Relaxation Techniques**: Practices such as meditation, deep breathing, and progressive muscle relaxation can help reduce stress and promote relaxation, which may enhance ACh activity and facilitate sleep onset.
4. **Dietary Considerations**: Consuming choline-rich foods, such as eggs, lean meats, and legumes, can support ACh synthesis. Additionally, magnesium-rich foods may help promote relaxation and improve sleep quality.
5. **Limiting Stimulants**: Reducing intake of caffeine and nicotine, especially in the hours leading up to bedtime, can improve sleep quality by minimizing their disruptive effects on ACh signaling.

Conclusion of Chapter 14

In summary, acetylcholine is a vital neurotransmitter that plays a crucial role in regulating sleep, particularly in the modulation of REM sleep and overall sleep architecture. Understanding ACh's involvement in sleep can inform both pharmacological and lifestyle interventions aimed at improving sleep quality and cognitive health.

As we proceed through this book, we will explore the fascinating connections between acetylcholine and the immune system, highlighting the broader implications of ACh in health and disease. This knowledge will further empower individuals to master acetylcholine production and availability for optimal overall well-being.

Chapter 15: Acetylcholine in the Immune System
Exploring the Link Between ACh and Immune Response

Acetylcholine (ACh) is predominantly recognized for its roles in the nervous system, particularly in neurotransmission, cognition, and muscle function. However, emerging research has illuminated the significant role that ACh plays in the immune system, revealing a fascinating interplay between cholinergic signaling and immune responses. This connection forms the basis of a field known as neuroimmunology, which explores how the nervous system and immune system interact.

1. **Cholinergic Innervation of Immune Organs**: Cholinergic neurons are found in various immune tissues, including the spleen and thymus. These neurons release ACh, which can influence immune cell activity. ACh acts on immune cells through nicotinic and muscarinic receptors, modulating their functions. For instance, T cells, macrophages, and dendritic cells express cholinergic receptors, indicating that they can respond to ACh.

2. **The Anti-Inflammatory Role of ACh**: ACh is increasingly recognized for its role in regulating inflammation. Activation of the vagus nerve, which releases ACh, can inhibit the production of pro-inflammatory cytokines. This mechanism is part of the "cholinergic anti-inflammatory pathway," which helps maintain homeostasis in the body during inflammatory responses. By modulating immune activity, ACh contributes to preventing excessive inflammation, which is critical for protecting tissues and organs.

3. **Implications for Autoimmune Disorders**: Dysregulation of cholinergic signaling may contribute to the pathophysiology of autoimmune diseases, where the immune system mistakenly attacks the body's tissues. For example, in conditions like rheumatoid arthritis and multiple sclerosis, ACh levels and receptor sensitivity can be altered. Understanding the cholinergic system's role in these diseases could open new avenues for therapeutic interventions that aim to restore balance to immune function.

Neuroimmunology examines the intricate relationship between the nervous and immune systems. This interdisciplinary field has gained traction in recent years, highlighting how the brain can influence immune responses and vice versa.

1. **Bidirectional Communication**: The communication between the nervous and immune systems is bidirectional. While neurotransmitters like ACh can influence immune cell behavior, immune signals can also affect neuronal function. Pro-inflammatory cytokines can alter neurotransmitter release and receptor sensitivity, leading to changes in mood, cognition, and behavior. This dynamic interaction underscores the complexity of health and disease.

2. **Stress and Immune Function**: Stress is known to impact both ACh levels and immune responses. Chronic stress can lead to increased sympathetic nervous system activity, resulting in the release of stress hormones that may suppress ACh signaling and promote inflammation. This relationship suggests that managing stress through techniques such as mindfulness and relaxation could benefit both cholinergic function and immune health.

3. **Potential Therapeutic Approaches**: The understanding of ACh's role in the immune system opens new therapeutic avenues. For instance, therapies that enhance cholinergic signaling could be explored as anti-inflammatory treatments. Similarly, agents that modulate the vagus nerve's activity might provide novel strategies for managing autoimmune and inflammatory conditions.

Conclusion of Chapter 15

In conclusion, the emerging understanding of acetylcholine's role in the immune system emphasizes the importance of this neurotransmitter beyond traditional neurological functions. ACh's involvement in immune regulation, inflammation, and neuroimmunology highlights the intricate connections between the nervous system and immune responses.

As we advance through this book, we will explore the role of acetylcholine in pain management, examining its influence on pain perception and potential therapeutic strategies that leverage cholinergic signaling. This exploration will further enhance our understanding of how to master acetylcholine production and availability for improved overall health and well-being.

Chapter 16: Acetylcholine in Pain Management
The Role of ACh in Pain Perception and Modulation

Acetylcholine (ACh) is not only crucial for cognitive function and muscle control but also plays a significant role in the modulation of pain. The complex interplay between the cholinergic system and pain pathways highlights ACh's potential as a target for pain management strategies.

1. **Cholinergic Mechanisms in Pain Perception**: ACh is involved in both the transmission and modulation of pain signals in the central and peripheral nervous systems. In the spinal cord, ACh can facilitate pain transmission through its action on nicotinic receptors located on nociceptive neurons (pain receptors). This facilitation can enhance the perception of pain.

2. **Inhibitory Effects**: Conversely, ACh also has inhibitory effects on pain pathways. It can act on muscarinic receptors, which are present in various brain regions involved in pain processing, such as the thalamus and cortex. Activation of these receptors can lead to analgesic effects, reducing the perception of pain and altering pain-related behavior.

3. **The Cholinergic Anti-Inflammatory Pathway**: ACh's role in the cholinergic anti-inflammatory pathway is particularly relevant in the context of pain management. The vagus nerve, when stimulated, releases ACh, which can inhibit the production of pro-inflammatory cytokines. This mechanism is important because many chronic pain conditions are associated with inflammation. By reducing inflammation through cholinergic signaling, ACh can help alleviate pain symptoms.

Potential Therapeutic Strategies Targeting ACh

Given the dual role of ACh in both facilitating and inhibiting pain perception, several therapeutic strategies could be considered to harness its effects for pain management.

1. **Cholinergic Agonists**: Drugs that stimulate cholinergic receptors, particularly muscarinic receptors, could be explored as potential analgesics. By enhancing ACh activity in pain-processing areas, these agents might reduce pain perception and improve pain management in conditions such as neuropathic pain or chronic inflammatory pain.

2. **Acetylcholinesterase Inhibitors**: As discussed in previous chapters, acetylcholinesterase inhibitors (AChEIs) prevent the breakdown of ACh, thereby increasing its availability at synapses. This increase could enhance the inhibitory effects of ACh on pain transmission and promote analgesia. Research into the use of AChEIs for pain management is ongoing, with promising results in some clinical trials.

3. **Neuromodulation Techniques**: Emerging neuromodulation techniques, such as transcutaneous electrical nerve stimulation (TENS) or vagus nerve stimulation (VNS), may leverage cholinergic pathways to alleviate pain. These techniques can enhance ACh release and modulate pain signals at various levels of the nervous system.

4. **Mind-Body Interventions**: Practices that promote relaxation and reduce stress, such as mindfulness meditation or yoga, may also enhance cholinergic signaling, providing a complementary approach to pain management. These interventions can stimulate the vagus nerve, promoting ACh release and reducing the perception of pain.

Implications for Chronic Pain Conditions

The understanding of ACh's role in pain modulation has significant implications for managing chronic pain conditions, including:

- **Neuropathic Pain**: Conditions such as diabetic neuropathy or postherpetic neuralgia may benefit from treatments targeting cholinergic signaling. Enhancing ACh activity could help alleviate the abnormal pain signals characteristic of these conditions.
- **Arthritis and Inflammatory Pain**: Given ACh's anti-inflammatory properties, therapies aimed at boosting cholinergic signaling may provide relief for individuals suffering from arthritis or other inflammatory pain syndromes.
- **Fibromyalgia**: This condition, characterized by widespread pain and fatigue, may also be influenced by dysregulation of the cholinergic system. Strategies to enhance ACh function could support overall pain management in these patients.

Conclusion of Chapter 16

In conclusion, acetylcholine plays a multifaceted role in pain perception and modulation. By understanding the mechanisms through which ACh influences pain pathways, we can explore various therapeutic strategies to improve pain management.

As we progress through this book, we will examine lifestyle factors that influence acetylcholine levels, emphasizing the importance of a holistic approach to mastering acetylcholine production and availability for overall health and well-being. This exploration will further underscore the interconnectedness of ACh with various physiological processes, including pain management and recovery.

Chapter 17: Lifestyle Factors Influencing Acetylcholine Levels

The Impact of Exercise, Stress, and Sleep on ACh Production

Acetylcholine (ACh) production and availability are significantly influenced by various lifestyle factors, including physical activity, stress management, and sleep quality. Understanding these influences can empower individuals to adopt practices that enhance ACh levels, thereby supporting cognitive function, emotional well-being, and overall health.

1. Exercise and Acetylcholine Levels

Regular physical activity has been consistently linked to improved cognitive function and enhanced cholinergic signaling. Exercise can positively impact ACh production through several mechanisms:

- **Increased Blood Flow**: Physical activity increases cerebral blood flow, delivering essential nutrients and oxygen to the brain. This improved circulation can support the synthesis and release of ACh in areas involved in memory and learning.
- **Neurogenesis and Plasticity**: Exercise promotes neurogenesis (the formation of new neurons) and synaptic plasticity, both of which are influenced by ACh. Increased levels of brain-derived neurotrophic factor (BDNF) during exercise can stimulate cholinergic function, enhancing ACh availability and its effects on cognitive processes.
- **Stress Reduction**: Regular exercise is an effective stress-reliever, which can mitigate the negative impact of stress hormones on cholinergic signaling. By lowering levels of cortisol and other stress-related hormones, exercise can help maintain optimal ACh production.
- **Endorphin Release**: Physical activity stimulates the release of endorphins and other neurotransmitters that can improve mood and cognitive function. This biochemical balance can support a healthy cholinergic system.

2. Stress Management and ACh Production

Stress has a profound impact on neurotransmitter systems, including the cholinergic system. Chronic stress can lead to dysregulation of ACh signaling and negatively affect cognitive function and emotional health. Strategies for managing stress are therefore crucial for supporting ACh levels:

- **Mindfulness and Meditation**: Mindfulness practices have been shown to reduce stress and promote relaxation. These practices can enhance cholinergic function by promoting the release of ACh, improving focus, and supporting emotional regulation.
- **Yoga and Tai Chi**: These mind-body practices combine physical movement, controlled breathing, and meditation, which can reduce stress and improve ACh levels. Regular participation in these activities has been associated with better mental health outcomes and enhanced cognitive function.
- **Breathing Exercises**: Deep, controlled breathing can activate the parasympathetic nervous system, promoting a state of calm and increasing ACh availability. Techniques such as diaphragmatic breathing can be particularly effective in reducing stress and enhancing relaxation.
- **Social Support**: Engaging in positive social interactions can buffer against stress and promote a sense of well-being. Supportive relationships can enhance resilience and potentially support healthy ACh levels through the reduction of stress.

3. The Role of Sleep in ACh Availability

Sleep is vital for cognitive health and is intricately connected to ACh production and signaling. ACh plays a critical role in regulating sleep cycles, particularly in the promotion of REM sleep. Here are ways sleep influences ACh levels:

- **REM Sleep and ACh**: ACh levels increase during REM sleep, facilitating this crucial stage of sleep associated with dreaming and memory consolidation. Quality REM sleep is essential for cognitive function, and disruptions can impair ACh signaling.
- **Sleep Quality and Cognitive Function**: Poor sleep quality can lead to decreased ACh availability, resulting in cognitive impairments, including memory deficits and reduced attention. Ensuring sufficient restorative sleep is essential for maintaining healthy ACh levels.
- **Circadian Rhythms**: The body's internal clock regulates the production of various neurotransmitters, including ACh. Establishing a consistent sleep routine helps maintain circadian rhythms, promoting optimal ACh production and overall brain health.
- **Sleep Hygiene Practices**: Implementing good sleep hygiene practices—such as creating a conducive sleep environment, limiting screen time before bed, and maintaining a regular sleep schedule—can support better sleep quality and subsequently enhance ACh levels.

Conclusion of Chapter 17

In conclusion, lifestyle factors such as exercise, stress management, and sleep quality significantly influence acetylcholine production and availability. By incorporating regular physical activity, practicing stress reduction techniques, and prioritizing restorative sleep, individuals can optimize their ACh levels and support cognitive and emotional health.

As we move forward in this book, we will delve into the connection between acetylcholine and neurodegeneration, exploring how ACh deficits contribute to diseases like Alzheimer's and potential interventions to preserve its function. This understanding will further reinforce the importance of mastering acetylcholine production and availability for overall well-being.

Chapter 18: Acetylcholine and Neurodegeneration
How ACh Deficits Contribute to Diseases Like Alzheimer's

Acetylcholine (ACh) has long been recognized for its critical role in cognitive function and memory formation. However, its decline is a prominent feature of several neurodegenerative diseases, particularly Alzheimer's disease (AD). Understanding the connection between ACh deficits and neurodegeneration provides insights into the mechanisms underlying these diseases and potential therapeutic strategies for intervention.

1. **The Role of ACh in Cognitive Function**: ACh is essential for various cognitive processes, including attention, learning, and memory consolidation. It facilitates communication between neurons and plays a vital role in synaptic plasticity, the mechanism through which synapses strengthen or weaken over time. A decline in ACh levels disrupts these processes, leading to cognitive impairments.

2. **Alzheimer's Disease and Cholinergic Dysfunction**: In Alzheimer's disease, one of the hallmark features is the loss of cholinergic neurons, particularly in the basal forebrain, which is crucial for ACh production. This degeneration results in significantly reduced ACh levels, contributing to the cognitive deficits observed in patients. The decline in ACh not only affects memory but also impairs the ability to learn new information and adapt to changes in the environment.

3. **Pathological Mechanisms**: The relationship between ACh deficits and Alzheimer's is also influenced by the disease's underlying pathological mechanisms, including amyloid-beta (Aβ) plaque formation and tau protein tangles. Aβ accumulation can disrupt cholinergic signaling, leading to further neuronal damage and loss. Additionally, neuroinflammation associated with Alzheimer's can exacerbate cholinergic dysfunction, creating a vicious cycle that accelerates cognitive decline.

Potential Interventions to Preserve ACh Function

Given the critical role of ACh in cognitive health, several therapeutic strategies are being explored to counteract ACh deficits in neurodegenerative diseases like Alzheimer's:

1. **Acetylcholinesterase Inhibitors (AChEIs)**: AChEIs are a cornerstone of Alzheimer's treatment. By inhibiting the enzyme that breaks down ACh, these drugs increase ACh levels in the brain, enhancing cholinergic signaling. Commonly prescribed AChEIs include donepezil, rivastigmine, and galantamine. These medications can provide symptomatic relief, improving cognitive function and quality of life for patients with Alzheimer's.

2. **Cholinergic Agonists**: Research is ongoing into the use of cholinergic agonists that stimulate ACh receptors directly. These agents may help restore cholinergic signaling in patients with neurodegenerative diseases and provide additional therapeutic options alongside AChEIs.

3. **Neuroprotective Strategies**: Interventions aimed at protecting cholinergic neurons from degeneration are crucial. This can include the use of antioxidants to combat oxidative stress, which is known to contribute to neuronal death in Alzheimer's. Lifestyle interventions such as regular physical exercise, a balanced diet rich in omega-3 fatty acids, and cognitive training may also support cholinergic health and protect against cognitive decline.

4. **Neuroinflammation Modulation**: Addressing neuroinflammation may help preserve cholinergic function. Research into anti-inflammatory agents that can target the inflammatory processes associated with Alzheimer's disease is ongoing. These strategies aim to reduce the neuroinflammatory response that contributes to cholinergic dysfunction.

5. **Gene Therapy and Biomarkers**: Advances in gene therapy offer promising avenues for targeting cholinergic dysfunction. Researchers are investigating methods to enhance the expression of choline acetyltransferase (ChAT), the enzyme responsible for ACh synthesis, in cholinergic neurons. Additionally, the identification of biomarkers for early cholinergic dysfunction could allow for earlier interventions in at-risk populations.

Conclusion of Chapter 18

In conclusion, acetylcholine deficits are a significant contributor to the cognitive impairments associated with neurodegenerative diseases like Alzheimer's. Understanding the intricate relationship between ACh and neurodegeneration opens up avenues for therapeutic intervention aimed at preserving cholinergic function and improving patient outcomes.

As we move forward in this book, we will explore the genetic factors influencing acetylcholine production, examining how genetic variations can affect ACh synthesis and availability. This exploration will further enhance our understanding of mastering acetylcholine production and availability for optimal cognitive health and well-being.

Chapter 19: Genetic Factors in Acetylcholine Production
Understanding Genetic Polymorphisms Affecting ACh Synthesis

The production and availability of acetylcholine (ACh) are influenced not only by lifestyle and environmental factors but also by genetic factors. Variations in genes that encode proteins involved in the synthesis, metabolism, and receptor signaling of ACh can significantly affect an individual's cholinergic function. Understanding these genetic influences is crucial for personalizing interventions aimed at optimizing ACh levels for cognitive and emotional health.

Genetic Variations in Cholinergic Pathways

- **Choline Acetyltransferase (ChAT)**: This enzyme is responsible for the synthesis of ACh from choline and acetyl-CoA. Variations in the CHAT gene can affect the enzyme's expression levels, potentially leading to altered ACh production and subsequent cognitive function.
- **Acetylcholinesterase (AChE)**: AChE is the enzyme that breaks down ACh in the synaptic cleft, thus regulating its availability. Genetic polymorphisms in the ACHE gene may influence ACh metabolism, impacting the cholinergic tone in the brain.
- **Nicotinic and Muscarinic Receptors**: Variations in genes encoding nicotinic (e.g., CHRNA5) and muscarinic receptors (e.g., CHRM2) can affect receptor function and density. These changes may alter an individual's response to cholinergic signaling, influencing cognitive processes and susceptibility to various neurodegenerative conditions.

The Role of Epigenetics in ACh Availability

In addition to genetic polymorphisms, epigenetic modifications can significantly influence ACh production and function. Epigenetics refers to changes in gene expression that do not involve alterations to the underlying DNA sequence, often resulting from environmental factors and lifestyle choices.

1. **Influence of Environment and Lifestyle**: Environmental factors, such as diet, stress, and exposure to toxins, can lead to epigenetic modifications that affect the expression of genes involved in cholinergic signaling. For example, a diet rich in choline can enhance the expression of genes related to ACh synthesis, whereas chronic stress may lead to epigenetic changes that impair ACh production.

2. **Methylation Patterns**: DNA methylation, a common epigenetic modification, can regulate the expression of genes involved in cholinergic pathways. For instance, hypermethylation of the CHAT gene may reduce its expression, leading to decreased ACh synthesis. Understanding these methylation patterns could provide insights into individual differences in ACh availability and related cognitive functions.

3. **Potential for Reversibility**: One of the exciting aspects of epigenetics is its potential for reversibility. Interventions such as dietary changes, exercise, and stress reduction may positively influence epigenetic marks, restoring optimal ACh levels and improving cognitive health. Research into the effects of lifestyle changes on epigenetic regulation of cholinergic pathways is an emerging area of interest.

Implications for Personalized Interventions

The understanding of genetic and epigenetic factors influencing ACh production offers a pathway for personalized interventions:

1. **Genetic Testing**: Genetic testing may help identify polymorphisms that affect ACh metabolism and signaling. Such information could guide personalized dietary and lifestyle recommendations aimed at optimizing ACh levels.
2. **Targeted Nutritional Interventions**: Individuals with specific genetic variations may benefit from tailored dietary strategies that enhance ACh synthesis. For example, those with polymorphisms associated with lower ChAT activity may require higher choline intake to support optimal ACh production.
3. **Lifestyle Modifications**: Epigenetic research suggests that lifestyle interventions can have a profound impact on ACh availability. Promoting stress management, physical activity, and cognitive engagement can lead to beneficial epigenetic changes that enhance cholinergic function.
4. **Pharmacogenomics**: Understanding genetic variations that influence individual responses to cholinergic medications can improve treatment outcomes for conditions related to ACh deficits, such as Alzheimer's disease or other cognitive disorders.

Conclusion of Chapter 19

In conclusion, genetic and epigenetic factors play a significant role in acetylcholine production and availability. Understanding these influences allows for the development of personalized strategies aimed at optimizing cholinergic function, which is crucial for cognitive health and overall well-being.

As we continue through this book, we will explore the future of acetylcholine research, focusing on emerging studies and potential breakthroughs that could shape our understanding and treatment of cholinergic dysfunction. This exploration will further enhance our ability to master acetylcholine production and availability for improved health outcomes.

Chapter 20: The Future of Acetylcholine Research
Emerging Studies and Potential Breakthroughs

The study of acetylcholine (ACh) has evolved significantly over the past few decades, revealing its crucial roles not only in the nervous system but also in other physiological processes, including immune function and pain modulation. As research progresses, new insights into ACh's multifaceted roles are emerging, paving the way for innovative therapies and interventions. This chapter explores the current landscape of ACh research, highlighting key areas of focus and potential breakthroughs.

Novel Therapeutics Targeting Cholinergic Pathways

- Recent studies are exploring novel compounds that target ACh receptors, aiming to enhance their efficacy and specificity. For instance, new cholinergic agonists are being developed that could selectively activate nicotinic or muscarinic receptors, leading to better-targeted treatments for cognitive disorders and neurodegenerative diseases.
- The exploration of AChE inhibitors has expanded beyond traditional uses, with ongoing research into their application for other conditions, such as chronic pain and depression. These studies aim to determine optimal dosages and treatment regimens for maximizing therapeutic effects while minimizing side effects.

Genetic and Epigenetic Research

- Advancements in genetic research are uncovering how genetic polymorphisms affect individual responses to cholinergic drugs and influence ACh levels. Understanding these genetic factors can lead to personalized medicine approaches that tailor treatments based on a patient's genetic profile.
- Epigenetic studies are revealing how lifestyle factors can influence ACh production and signaling. Future research may focus on identifying specific epigenetic modifications that enhance cholinergic function, offering potential therapeutic targets for intervention.

Neuroimmunology and ACh

The emerging field of neuroimmunology has highlighted the connection between ACh and immune responses, suggesting new avenues for treating autoimmune disorders and chronic inflammatory conditions. Future research will likely focus on the therapeutic potential of modulating cholinergic signaling to regulate inflammation and improve immune function.

Role of ACh in Neurodegenerative Diseases

Ongoing research is investigating the role of ACh in other neurodegenerative diseases beyond Alzheimer's, such as Parkinson's disease and Huntington's disease. Understanding how ACh deficits contribute to these conditions may lead to novel therapeutic strategies that address cognitive and motor symptoms.

Exploration of ACh in Mental Health

Studies are increasingly examining the relationship between ACh and mental health conditions, including anxiety and depression. Research focusing on how ACh signaling influences mood regulation may lead to innovative treatment options that target the cholinergic system for improving mental health outcomes.

Innovations in Treatments Targeting ACh Pathways

As the understanding of ACh's roles expands, innovative treatment strategies are being developed:

Combining Pharmacological and Behavioral Interventions

Research is exploring the combined effects of pharmacological agents that enhance ACh availability with behavioral interventions, such as cognitive training and mindfulness practices. This integrative approach may yield greater improvements in cognitive function and emotional well-being.

Use of Biomarkers

The identification of biomarkers related to ACh signaling may facilitate the early detection of cholinergic dysfunction. Biomarker-guided interventions could lead to earlier and more targeted treatments for cognitive decline and neurodegenerative diseases.

Advanced Drug Delivery Systems

Innovations in drug delivery systems, such as nanoparticles and targeted delivery methods, are being researched to improve the efficacy of cholinergic therapies. These systems aim to enhance the specificity and bioavailability of drugs targeting the cholinergic system.

Neurofeedback and Biofeedback Techniques

Emerging neurofeedback techniques that train individuals to enhance ACh-related brain activity may provide non-invasive methods for improving cognitive function and emotional regulation. Research in this area could offer new tools for personal development and mental health management.

Exploration of the Gut-Brain Axis

The relationship between gut health and brain function is a growing area of interest. Research on how gut microbiota influence ACh production and signaling may uncover novel therapeutic approaches for enhancing cognitive function through dietary interventions.

Conclusion of Chapter 20

In conclusion, the future of acetylcholine research is promising, with emerging studies and innovations poised to enhance our understanding of ACh's multifaceted roles in health and disease. By leveraging advances in genetics, pharmacology, and neuroimmunology, researchers are paving the way for new therapeutic strategies that could significantly impact the management of cognitive disorders, mental health conditions, and neurodegenerative diseases.

As we continue through this book, we will examine real-life case studies in acetylcholine research, focusing on practical applications and the lessons learned from clinical settings. This exploration will provide insights into the implementation of ACh-related findings in everyday life and further enhance our understanding of mastering acetylcholine production and availability for optimal health outcomes.

Chapter 21: Case Studies in Acetylcholine Research
Real-Life Examples of ACh Manipulation in Clinical Settings

The study of acetylcholine (ACh) has yielded numerous insights into its vital role in health and disease, particularly through various case studies. These real-life examples illustrate the practical applications of ACh research, showcasing how manipulations of ACh pathways have informed clinical practice and improved patient outcomes. This chapter highlights several significant case studies that provide valuable lessons in understanding and mastering ACh production and availability.

Case Study 1: The Use of Acetylcholinesterase Inhibitors in Alzheimer's Disease

- **Background**: Alzheimer's disease is characterized by significant cholinergic dysfunction, with decreased levels of ACh due to the degeneration of cholinergic neurons. AChE inhibitors like donepezil and rivastigmine are commonly prescribed to enhance ACh availability in the brain.
- **Findings**: In clinical trials, patients receiving AChE inhibitors showed improvements in cognitive function and quality of life compared to those receiving placebo treatments. The studies highlighted the importance of timely intervention, showing that earlier initiation of treatment could lead to more substantial cognitive benefits.
- **Lessons Learned**: This case underscores the need for early diagnosis and intervention in Alzheimer's disease and the potential of pharmacological strategies to enhance cholinergic function and mitigate cognitive decline.

Case Study 2: Cholinergic Modulation in Parkinson's Disease

- **Background**: In Parkinson's disease, there is not only a loss of dopaminergic neurons but also alterations in cholinergic function. Some patients experience cognitive and mood disturbances alongside motor symptoms, which can be exacerbated by cholinergic deficits.
- **Findings**: A clinical study involving patients with Parkinson's utilized a combination of dopaminergic therapies and muscarinic receptor agonists. The results indicated improvements in both motor and cognitive symptoms, suggesting that cholinergic modulation could be beneficial for comprehensive management of Parkinson's.
- **Lessons Learned**: This case illustrates the value of a multi-targeted approach in treating neurodegenerative diseases, where addressing both dopaminergic and cholinergic systems can lead to improved outcomes for patients.

Case Study 3: The Impact of Dietary Choline on Cognitive Performance

- **Background**: Choline is a vital nutrient for ACh synthesis, and dietary intake can influence cognitive health. A study explored the effects of choline supplementation on cognitive performance in older adults.
- **Findings**: Participants who received choline supplements demonstrated enhanced memory performance and improved scores on cognitive assessments compared to a control group. Brain imaging revealed increased activity in regions associated with memory and learning.
- **Lessons Learned**: This case emphasizes the importance of nutrition in supporting cholinergic function and cognitive health, highlighting dietary interventions as a potential strategy for enhancing ACh production and availability.

Case Study 4: Cholinergic Dysfunction in Depression

- **Background**: Research has increasingly linked cholinergic dysfunction to mood disorders, including depression. A clinical trial investigated the effects of cholinergic agonists on depressive symptoms in patients with treatment-resistant depression.
- **Findings**: The study found that administration of a specific cholinergic agonist led to significant reductions in depressive symptoms for many participants, suggesting a novel pathway for treatment.
- **Lessons Learned**: This case highlights the potential of targeting cholinergic pathways in the treatment of mood disorders, opening new avenues for therapy in populations who have not responded to traditional antidepressants.

Case Study 5: The Role of Physical Activity in Enhancing ACh Availability

- **Background**: Regular physical activity has been shown to promote neurogenesis and improve cognitive function. A study investigated the effects of an exercise program on ACh levels and cognitive performance in older adults.
- **Findings**: Participants who engaged in regular aerobic exercise showed significant increases in ACh levels, accompanied by improvements in memory and cognitive flexibility. The results underscored the link between physical activity and cholinergic health.
- **Lessons Learned**: This case illustrates the critical role of lifestyle factors, such as exercise, in enhancing ACh production and overall cognitive health, reinforcing the importance of a holistic approach to managing cholinergic function.

Conclusion of Chapter 21

The case studies presented in this chapter provide compelling evidence of the critical role of acetylcholine in various health conditions. By manipulating ACh pathways through pharmacological, dietary, and lifestyle interventions, researchers and clinicians can enhance cognitive function, improve emotional well-being, and potentially alter the course of neurodegenerative diseases.

As we proceed to the next chapter, we will explore practical applications of acetylcholine mastery, focusing on how to implement findings from research into daily life to maintain optimal ACh levels for better health outcomes. This exploration will further empower individuals to take charge of their cholinergic health through informed choices and strategies.

Chapter 22: Practical Applications of Acetylcholine Mastery

How to Implement Findings into Daily Life

Mastering acetylcholine production and availability is essential for optimizing cognitive function, emotional health, and overall well-being. This chapter provides practical strategies to apply the insights gained from previous chapters, enabling individuals to enhance their cholinergic function through lifestyle modifications, dietary choices, and other interventions.

1. Nutritional Strategies

Increase Choline Intake

- Eggs (particularly the yolk)
- Liver and other organ meats
- Fish and poultry
- Dairy products
- Cruciferous vegetables (e.g., broccoli, Brussels sprouts)
- Nuts and seeds
- Whole grains

- **Consider Supplements**: For those who struggle to meet their choline needs through diet alone, supplements such as phosphatidylcholine or choline bitartrate can be beneficial. However, it's essential to consult with a healthcare professional before starting any supplementation regimen.
- **Emphasize Omega-3 Fatty Acids**: Omega-3s support neuronal health and may enhance ACh receptor function. Incorporate sources like fatty fish (salmon, mackerel), walnuts, flaxseeds, and chia seeds into your diet.
- **Antioxidant-Rich Foods**: Consume fruits and vegetables high in antioxidants, such as berries, leafy greens, and nuts, to combat oxidative stress, which can impair cholinergic function.

2. Lifestyle Modifications

- **Regular Physical Activity**: Engaging in regular aerobic exercise has been shown to enhance ACh production and improve cognitive function. Aim for at least 150 minutes of moderate-intensity exercise per week, incorporating activities like walking, cycling, swimming, or dancing.
- **Stress Management Techniques**: Chronic stress can negatively affect ACh levels. Practice stress-reduction strategies such as:

- Mindfulness meditation
- Deep breathing exercises
- Yoga or tai chi
- Engaging in hobbies and activities that promote relaxation

Prioritize Sleep Hygiene

- Maintaining a consistent sleep schedule
- Creating a comfortable sleep environment (dark, quiet, and cool)
- Limiting screen time before bed
- Practicing relaxation techniques before sleep

3. Cognitive Engagement

- **Mental Stimulation**: Engage in activities that challenge the brain, such as puzzles, reading, learning new skills, or playing musical instruments. These activities can enhance neuroplasticity and support cholinergic function.
- **Social Interaction**: Foster social connections and engage in meaningful conversations. Social interaction is linked to better cognitive health and can help maintain ACh levels.

4. Pharmacological Considerations

- **Discuss Medications with Healthcare Providers**: If you are experiencing cognitive decline or related symptoms, consult a healthcare professional about the potential benefits of cholinergic medications or supplements. Personalized medication management can help optimize ACh availability.
- **Monitor Cholinergic Drug Effects**: For those already on cholinergic medications, keeping track of any changes in cognitive function, mood, or overall well-being is crucial. Regular follow-ups with healthcare providers can help adjust dosages or explore alternative treatments as needed.

5. Continuous Education and Awareness

- **Stay Informed**: Keep up-to-date with the latest research on ACh and its role in health. Engaging with credible sources, such as scientific journals, health organizations, and reputable websites, can provide valuable insights into new developments.
- **Participate in Workshops and Seminars**: Attend events focused on cognitive health, nutrition, and wellness to learn more about practical applications of ACh mastery. Engaging with experts can deepen your understanding and provide new strategies for implementation.

Conclusion of Chapter 22

Mastering acetylcholine production and availability involves a multifaceted approach that combines dietary strategies, lifestyle modifications, cognitive engagement, and potential pharmacological interventions. By implementing these practical applications into daily life, individuals can enhance their cholinergic function, supporting cognitive health and emotional well-being.

As we move to the next chapter, we will discuss the challenges faced in acetylcholine research, addressing misconceptions, ethical considerations, and the obstacles researchers encounter in their pursuit of knowledge and advancements in cholinergic therapies. This discussion will further enrich our understanding of the complexities surrounding ACh and its role in health and disease.

Chapter 23: Overcoming Challenges in Acetylcholine Research

Addressing Common Misconceptions and Hurdles

The field of acetylcholine (ACh) research presents numerous opportunities for advancing our understanding of its role in health and disease. However, it also faces several challenges, including misconceptions, methodological hurdles, and ethical considerations. This chapter aims to address these issues to pave the way for more effective research and application of ACh knowledge.

1. Common Misconceptions

- **Misconception: ACh is only important for memory and learning**

    While ACh is well-known for its role in cognitive processes, particularly memory and learning, its functions extend beyond the brain. ACh is critical in muscle contraction, autonomic nervous system regulation, and immune response. Recognizing the widespread influence of ACh can help direct research towards understanding its roles in various physiological systems.

- **Misconception: AChE inhibitors are only for Alzheimer's disease**

    Although acetylcholinesterase (AChE) inhibitors are prominently used in treating Alzheimer's disease, they also have potential applications in other conditions, including Parkinson's disease and certain mood disorders. This narrow view can limit exploration into the broader therapeutic benefits of cholinergic modulation.

- **Misconception: Cholinergic dysfunction is solely a consequence of aging**

    While age-related decline in ACh production is a significant factor in cognitive decline, cholinergic dysfunction can occur in younger populations due to factors such as stress, poor nutrition, and genetic predispositions. This misconception can hinder early interventions that could benefit younger individuals at risk for cognitive impairments.

2. Methodological Hurdles

- **Research Design Limitations**

    Many studies on ACh focus narrowly on specific diseases or conditions, often failing to consider the broader context of cholinergic function across multiple systems. Future research should adopt multidisciplinary approaches that explore the interactions between ACh and other neurotransmitter systems, lifestyle factors, and environmental influences.

- **Individual Variability**

    The effects of ACh can vary significantly among individuals due to genetic differences, health status, and lifestyle choices. This variability can complicate research findings and clinical applications. Employing personalized medicine approaches and stratifying study populations based on genetic and phenotypic characteristics may help address this challenge.

- **Measurement Challenges**

    Accurately measuring ACh levels and receptor activity in vivo remains a significant challenge. Current methodologies may not capture the dynamic nature of ACh signaling effectively. Advances in imaging techniques and biomarker identification are necessary to improve our understanding of ACh's role in real-time physiological processes.

3. Ethical Considerations

- **Informed Consent in Clinical Trials**

    Research involving cholinergic drugs, particularly in vulnerable populations such as those with cognitive impairments, raises ethical concerns regarding informed consent. Researchers must ensure that participants fully understand the potential risks and benefits of participation and are capable of making informed decisions.

- **Long-Term Effects of Cholinergic Modulation**

    The long-term consequences of manipulating ACh levels through pharmacological interventions remain largely unknown. Continuous monitoring and follow-up studies are essential to assess the safety and efficacy of these interventions, especially for chronic use.

- **Equity in Research Access**

    Ensuring equitable access to cholinergic treatments and participation in clinical trials is vital. Historically, marginalized populations may have been underrepresented in research, which can lead to disparities in treatment efficacy and outcomes. Efforts should focus on inclusivity and addressing barriers to participation in ACh-related studies.

4. Moving Forward

To overcome these challenges, the following strategies can be employed:

- **Collaborative Research Initiatives**

    Encouraging collaborations among neuroscientists, pharmacologists, nutritionists, and clinicians can foster a more comprehensive understanding of ACh. Multi-disciplinary research initiatives can lead to innovative approaches for studying ACh's diverse roles in health and disease.

- **Public Education and Awareness**

    Increasing public understanding of the importance of ACh beyond cognitive function can help reduce misconceptions. Educational initiatives can empower individuals to engage in proactive health measures that support cholinergic function.

- **Advancing Research Technologies**

    Investing in new technologies for measuring ACh dynamics, such as advanced imaging techniques and biomarker discovery, can provide deeper insights into cholinergic signaling and its implications for health.

Conclusion of Chapter 23

Overcoming the challenges in acetylcholine research is essential for unlocking its full potential in enhancing health outcomes. By addressing misconceptions, refining research methodologies, and considering ethical implications, we can foster a more robust understanding of ACh's multifaceted roles in the body.

In the next chapter, we will summarize key concepts and findings from this book, exploring future research trajectories and the unanswered questions that remain in the field of acetylcholine mastery. This will provide a comprehensive overview of the advancements made and the pathways for future exploration in this vital area of health science.

Chapter 24: Summary and Future Directions
Recap of Key Concepts and Findings

As we approach the conclusion of our exploration into mastering acetylcholine (ACh) production and availability, it is crucial to summarize the key concepts and findings that have emerged throughout this book. Understanding ACh's multifaceted role in the body provides a foundation for both theoretical knowledge and practical applications aimed at enhancing cognitive health and overall well-being.

1. **Significance of Acetylcholine**:

   Acetylcholine is a pivotal neurotransmitter involved in various physiological functions, including muscle contraction, cognitive processes, and the modulation of the autonomic nervous system. Its importance extends beyond the central nervous system to include peripheral functions that affect everything from movement to mood regulation.

2. **Neurotransmission and Receptor Function**:

   ACh operates through two primary types of receptors: nicotinic and muscarinic. Understanding how these receptors function and their distribution across different body systems has illuminated pathways through which ACh affects both neurological and muscular responses.

3. **Synthesis and Production**:

   The synthesis of ACh involves critical enzymes such as choline acetyltransferase and acetylcholinesterase. Factors influencing ACh production include nutritional sources of choline, genetic variations, and lifestyle choices. A balanced diet and appropriate supplementation can enhance ACh availability and, consequently, its physiological effects.

4. **Role in Cognitive Function**:

   ACh has a profound impact on cognitive functions, particularly memory and learning. Research has established a clear link between ACh levels and neuroplasticity, highlighting its potential as a therapeutic target for cognitive enhancement and neurodegenerative diseases.

5. **Impact of Aging and Neurodegeneration**:

    Aging is associated with a decline in ACh production, contributing to cognitive impairments and neurodegenerative diseases such as Alzheimer's. Recognizing these changes allows for early intervention strategies aimed at preserving cognitive function through dietary, lifestyle, and pharmacological means.

6. **Mental Health Connections**:

    ACh levels are intricately linked to mood and emotional regulation. Understanding this connection has opened new avenues for treating mood disorders, including the potential use of cholinergic agents to improve mood and reduce anxiety.

7. **Lifestyle Influences**:

    Physical activity, stress management, and sleep quality are all critical factors influencing ACh levels. Strategies that promote a healthy lifestyle can support optimal cholinergic function, enhancing both cognitive and physical health.

8. **Research Challenges and Ethical Considerations**:

    The chapter on overcoming challenges highlighted misconceptions, methodological hurdles, and ethical considerations in ACh research. Addressing these issues is essential for advancing knowledge and ensuring the safe application of findings in clinical settings.

Future Research Trajectories

Looking forward, several promising areas of research can enhance our understanding and application of ACh:

1. **Personalized Medicine**:

   As research progresses, the ability to tailor treatments based on individual genetic and phenotypic profiles will become increasingly important. Understanding genetic polymorphisms affecting ACh synthesis can lead to personalized approaches in treating cognitive and mood disorders.

2. **Innovative Therapeutics**:

   Continued exploration of cholinergic drugs, including AChE inhibitors and novel compounds targeting specific receptors, may yield new therapeutic strategies for conditions linked to cholinergic dysfunction.

3. **Dietary Interventions**:

   Research into dietary sources of choline and their impact on ACh levels could inform public health guidelines aimed at optimizing cognitive health across the lifespan. Longitudinal studies examining the effects of dietary choline intake on cognitive outcomes are particularly warranted.

4. **Integration of Neuroimmunology**:

   The emerging field of neuroimmunology, which explores the interplay between the nervous and immune systems, presents exciting opportunities to investigate how ACh modulates immune responses and how these interactions affect neurological health.

5. **Expanding Understanding of Neuroplasticity**:
   Further investigation into the mechanisms by which ACh influences synaptic plasticity can inform rehabilitation practices and cognitive enhancement strategies, particularly in populations recovering from injury or neurological illness.

Unanswered Questions

Despite the advancements made in ACh research, several critical questions remain:

- How do different forms of stress impact ACh production and receptor sensitivity?
- What are the long-term effects of chronic ACh manipulation through pharmacological interventions?
- How can we effectively measure and monitor ACh dynamics in real-time in vivo?
- What are the implications of ACh's role in neurodegenerative diseases for developing preventative strategies?

Conclusion of Chapter 24

In conclusion, mastering acetylcholine production and availability offers a pathway to enhancing cognitive health and addressing a range of neurological and psychological conditions. The insights gained from this comprehensive exploration provide a strong foundation for future research and practical applications. As we move forward, the integration of this knowledge into everyday practices can empower individuals to optimize their cholinergic function for improved health outcomes.

In the next chapter, we will summarize our findings and present final thoughts on the importance of continued education and exploration in mastering acetylcholine and its vast potential for enhancing human health.

Chapter 25: Conclusion: The Path Forward

As we conclude our comprehensive exploration of acetylcholine (ACh), its production, availability, and its vital role in various physiological processes, it is essential to reflect on the knowledge gained and the future direction of research and application in this field. Mastering acetylcholine production not only holds promise for advancing our understanding of the brain and body but also offers tangible strategies for improving health and well-being across the lifespan.

Summary of Key Takeaways

1. **Essential Role of ACh**:

    Throughout this book, we have established that acetylcholine is crucial not only for cognitive functions such as memory and learning but also for motor control, mood regulation, and even immune response. Its widespread effects underline the importance of maintaining optimal ACh levels for overall health.

2. **Multifaceted Factors Influencing ACh Levels**:

    We examined the various factors that influence ACh production, including nutritional sources, genetic predispositions, and lifestyle choices. This highlights the need for a holistic approach to health, considering how diet, exercise, stress management, and sleep can significantly impact cholinergic function.

3. **Emerging Research and Therapeutics**:

    The future of ACh research is promising, with ongoing studies exploring new therapeutic applications for cholinergic drugs, dietary interventions, and the potential for personalized medicine. Understanding genetic and epigenetic influences on ACh synthesis may lead to more effective treatments for neurodegenerative diseases, mood disorders, and cognitive impairments.

4. **Practical Applications**:

   The practical applications of our findings emphasize actionable strategies individuals can implement in their daily lives. From dietary choices rich in choline to lifestyle modifications that support overall brain health, empowering individuals to take charge of their cholinergic function can lead to improved cognitive and emotional outcomes.

5. **Addressing Challenges and Ethical Considerations**:

   We discussed the challenges in ACh research, including misconceptions, methodological hurdles, and ethical considerations. Moving forward, it is crucial to address these challenges through collaborative research, improved methodologies, and ethical transparency in clinical trials.

The Path Forward

The journey towards mastering acetylcholine production and availability does not end with this book. Instead, it serves as a springboard for continued exploration and innovation in the field of neuroscience and health sciences. Here are some considerations for the path ahead:

- **Encourage Continued Research**:

    As the understanding of ACh continues to evolve, researchers should be encouraged to pursue interdisciplinary studies that examine the interplay between ACh and other neurotransmitters, as well as its role in various diseases. Collaborative efforts across fields can yield new insights and foster innovative therapeutic strategies.

- **Promote Public Awareness**:

    Increasing public knowledge about the importance of ACh can lead to greater awareness of lifestyle factors that influence its production. Educational campaigns and community programs can empower individuals to make informed choices that promote cholinergic health.

- **Support Clinical Trials and Studies**:

    Participation in clinical trials should be encouraged to advance the understanding of ACh-related therapies. Individuals who qualify can contribute to the body of knowledge that informs best practices in treating conditions associated with cholinergic dysfunction.

- **Embrace Personalized Approaches**:

    The future of healthcare lies in personalized medicine. As more is learned about genetic variations affecting ACh synthesis, tailoring interventions to individual needs could maximize therapeutic efficacy and minimize adverse effects.

- **Foster an Ongoing Dialogue**:
    The conversation surrounding acetylcholine and its implications for health should remain dynamic. Continued discourse among scientists, healthcare professionals, and the public can drive innovation and enhance the collective understanding of this critical neurotransmitter.

Final Thoughts

Mastering acetylcholine production and availability is an ongoing endeavor that holds the potential to transform our approach to health, cognition, and emotional well-being. By synthesizing the knowledge presented in this book and remaining committed to further exploration, we can unlock new avenues for enhancing life quality and longevity. The path forward is not just about understanding acetylcholine; it is about leveraging this knowledge to create healthier, more fulfilling lives for ourselves and future generations.

Let us continue to seek knowledge, share insights, and apply what we learn to make a positive impact in the realm of health and beyond. Together, we can foster a future where the mastery of acetylcholine contributes to the enhancement of human potential and well-being.